EVERYTHING ABOUT

CALORIE CYCLING

DIET

Complete Nutritional Cookbook, Foods, Meal Plan, And Recipes To Help Adapt To Greater Weight Loss, Less Hunger, And Improved Ability

DR. ALVIN BRANTLEY

Disclaimer

The information provided in this book is intended for general informational purposes only. It is not a substitute for professional medical advice, diagnosis, or treatment.

You should not use the information in this book for diagnosing or treating a health problem or disease by self decision. Always seek the advice of your physician or other qualified health provider with any questions you may have regarding a medical condition.

The author and publisher of this book make no representations or warranties with respect to the accuracy, applicability, fitness, or completeness of the contents of this book. The information contained in this book is based on the author's research and experience, and it is shared with the understanding that the author is not engaged in rendering medical, health, or any other kind of professional advice for you by this book.

The author does not endorse or promote any specific products, brands, or companies related to the contents provided in this book.

Any mention of products or services in this book is for informational purposes only and does not constitute an endorsement.

The author has not entered into any affiliate marketing agreements and has not signed any endorsement deals with individuals, organizations, or companies.

Readers are encouraged to consult with their healthcare providers before making any dietary or lifestyle chaSnges based on the information provided in this book. The author and publisher disclaim any liability for the decisions made by readers based on the information in this book.

Contents

Dietary Cycling for Calories

Calorie cycling, often referred to as calorie shifting, is a dietary approach in which the amount of calories consumed is changed daily, weekly, or monthly. This strategy is based on the idea that the body cannot become accustomed to a steady calorie intake, which may result in plateaus in either muscle growth or weight loss. This article explores the specifics of the calorie cycling diet, including its advantages, methods for carrying it out, and how to combine it with exercise for the best outcomes.

Comprehending the Cycle of Calories

The idea behind calorie cycling is to vary the amount of calories consumed to maintain the body's metabolic flexibility. Calorie cycling alternates days with greater and lower caloric intake, in contrast to standard diets that set a set daily limit. This modification is thought to improve fat burning, speed up metabolism, and encourage better adherence to dietary plans.

The Advantages of Cycling Calorie

The ability of calorie cycling to thwart metabolic adaption is one of its main advantages. The body is less likely to adapt to a certain energy level when calories are consumed infrequently, which promotes more prolonged weight management success. Calorie cycling proponents also assert that it might aid in controlling appetite and metabolism-related hormones like ghrelin and leptin.

Putting Calorie Cycling Into Practice

Careful planning and calorie monitoring are necessary when implementing a calorie-cycling diet. The different techniques for calorie cycling that are covered in this section include weekly, monthly, and daily strategies. It explains how to set calorie targets for high and low days, highlighting the need to comprehend personal energy requirements and objectives.

CHAPTER ONE

Recognizing Calories

The basic unit of energy that the body obtains from food and drink is calories. These units are necessary for maintaining life, assisting with physiological processes, and supporting body functions.

To put it simply, knowing about calories is essential to understanding how our bodies use the energy that comes from the food we eat.

Fundamentals Of Energy And Calorie

The fundamentals of energy and calories entail exploring the idea that calories serve as the fuel for the body's daily functions.

Food's energy content is expressed in calories, and the energy content of the various macronutrients varies.

Proteins and carbohydrates have about 4 calories per gram, but fats have 9 calories per gram, making them a more concentrated source of energy.

The foundation for comprehending the function of calories in nutrition is this basic knowledge.

The Value Of Energy Consumption

The direct effect that caloric consumption has on general health and well-being makes it significant.

Maintaining healthy bodily functions, such as metabolism, cell repair, and the regulation of vital processes, depends on the body getting the energy it needs.

A sufficient intake of calories guarantees that the body gets the nutrients it needs for optimum performance and maintains energy levels for daily tasks.

The Impact Of Calories On Weight

A key factor in managing weight is calorie intake since body weight is determined by the ratio of calories burned to calories consumed.

People acquire weight when they eat more calories than their bodies need because the extra energy is deposited as fat.

On the other hand, weight loss occurs when there is a calorie deficit—that is when the body uses more energy than it takes in. It is essential for everyone trying to effectively manage their weight to comprehend this dynamic.

Frequently Held Myths Regarding Calories

The idea of calories is surrounded by several myths, which further obscures sensible dietary guidelines.

The common misperception is that calories are calories regardless of where they come from.

In actuality, the caliber of the calories is important because different foods have different effects on general wellness.

The idea that cutting calories dramatically is the best approach to losing weight is another common fallacy.

This oversimplification can be harmful to one's health and ignores the significance of eating a balanced diet. It is essential to debunk these widespread myths to promote a more sophisticated understanding of calorie consumption.

CHAPTER TWO

The Mechanism Of Calorie Cycling

Calorie cycling, sometimes referred to as calorie shifting or cyclical dieting, is a weekly or daily calorie intake method.

In contrast to conventional, static calorie regimens, this strategy seeks to enhance metabolic processes for better overall health and weight management.

Calorie cycling research focuses on controlling energy intake to maintain physical flexibility and avoid metabolic adaption, which frequently happens with extended calorie restriction.

Cycling Of Calories And Metabolism

A key factor in the success of the calorie-cycling diet is metabolism. The body uses a complicated series of molecular reactions called metabolism to turn food into energy.

Calorie cycling aims to prevent the body from becoming accustomed to a regularly low-calorie diet, therefore preventing the metabolism from slowing down.

Changes in the amount of calories consumed can increase metabolic rate, which may aid in fat loss and maintain lean muscle mass.

The Function Of Hormones In Calorie Cycling

Hormones have a major impact on how the body stores and burns fat, as well as controlling metabolism.

Insulin, leptin, and ghrelin levels are among the hormones that are significantly impacted by calorie cycling. Hormonal variations have the potential to impact the body's tendency to store or release fat, as well as appetite and satiety.

Through deliberate modifications of their caloric intake, those who engage in calorie cycling seek to manipulate these hormones in a way that promotes increased thermogenesis.

The Impact Of Cycling Calories On Body Composition

A major objective of calorie cycling is to positively impact body composition. People may lose less lean muscle mass while losing more fat if they alternate between higher and lower calorie consumption intervals.

The deliberate manipulation of calories is intended to produce a deficit in calories during some stages of the diet while permitting maintenance or even a small excess during other stages.

This strategy is supposed to encourage fat loss without inducing the metabolic changes that frequently come with extended calorie restriction.

Investigations And Analysis Of Calorie Cycling

Calorie cycling has been the subject of numerous research comparing its efficacy to typical continuous calorie restriction. Calorie cycling may be beneficial for weight loss, fat removal, and metabolic rate, according to research.

Studies suggest that this method, which offers sporadic release from dietary restrictions, may be more sustainable for long-term adherence than rigorous calorie restriction.

To completely comprehend the physiological processes and long-term effects of calorie cycling for various groups, more study is necessary.

The science underlying calorie cycling includes a thorough comprehension of hormone control, metabolism, and how these factors interact to affect body composition.

It is critical to take into account the various reactions and possible advantages based on scientific data when people investigate this dietary approach.

We will probably continue to refine our understanding of calorie cycling and how it supports long-term, healthy weight management.

CHAPTER THREE

Settlement For Calorie Cycling

Calorie shifting, or calorie cycling, is a dietary approach in which the number of calories consumed is changed either weekly or daily.

Its purpose is to keep the body from adjusting to a steady calorie intake, which may accelerate weight reduction and improve metabolic efficiency.

Understanding the underlying ideas and variables is essential before beginning calorie cycling.

Evaluating Your Present Diet

Evaluating your existing eating patterns is the first step in implementing a calorie-cycling diet.

This entails maintaining an extensive food journal to monitor daily caloric consumption and the distribution of macronutrients.

A better understanding of the nutritional makeup of your meals enables you to approach calorie cycling with greater knowledge.

Furthermore, determining any unhealthful eating habits or nutritional deficits might assist in customizing the calorie cycling program to meet certain dietary requirements.

Creating Calorie Objectives

Clearly defined caloric targets are necessary for the successful use of calorie cycling.

This involves figuring out how many calories you need each day depending on your age, gender, activity level, and goals for weight loss or maintenance.

Setting calorie targets is the first step toward designing a cycling schedule that will help you achieve your goals.

A successful calorie cycling technique requires striking a balance between providing dietary requirements and creating an energy deficit for weight loss.

Selecting The Appropriate Cycling Sequence

There are numerous calorie cycling patterns available, each with a distinct layout.

Frequent patterns include weekly cycles, which alternate higher and lower calorie days throughout the week, and daily calorie variations, which involve alternating between high and low days of eating.

The pattern selected will rely on lifestyle choices, exercise objectives, and personal preferences.

While some might find weekly planning more flexible, others might find daily swings easier to handle.

Organizing Your Meals

Meal planning comes next once you've selected a cycling pattern and established your calorie objectives. It is essential to strategically distribute calories throughout the cycle to maximize energy and nutrient intake.

To satisfy nutritional requirements, concentrate on including nutrient-dense foods on days with increased caloric intake.

Prioritize lean meats, veggies high in fiber, and healthy fats on days when you're cutting calories to ensure that you're getting enough nutrients and staying full. Planning and preparing meals in advance is crucial to maintaining the calorie cycling method.

Beginning a calorie-cycling diet requires a thorough strategy that includes evaluating your existing diet, establishing attainable calorie targets, selecting a suitable cycle pattern, and scheduling meals appropriately.

You can take full advantage of the potential health and weight management benefits of calorie cycling by implementing these steps into your eating strategy.

Calorie Cycling Types

There are various variations of calorie cycling, and each one has a different strategy for adjusting caloric intake. Calorie cycling on a daily, weekly, and monthly basis is one such classification.

The Cycle Of Daily Calories

Daily calorie cycling is the practice of switching up the number of high- and low-calorie days in a given week.

On high-calorie days, people eat more calories than they usually do, and on low-calorie days, they eat fewer calories.

By generating a weekly caloric deficit, this cyclical pattern seeks to promote fat reduction without causing the metabolic adaption that comes with continuous calorie restriction.

Weekly Cycling Of Calories

The cyclical strategy is extended over a longer period with weekly calorie cycling. According to this concept, people might consume more calories for a few days in a row before cutting back on those calories for a few days.

Weekly cycling's flexibility makes it possible to plan more strategically and accommodate social occasions or changes in activity levels. Those who like a less rigid structure may find this method especially appealing.

Monthly Cycle Of Calories

A longer-term approach is used in monthly calorie cycling, which alternates between periods of increased and decreased calorie consumption over a month.

This strategy might work for people who would rather have longer stretches of stability interspersed with shorter bursts of more substantial calorie changes. Cycling once a month can offer flexibility and the advantages of calorie shifting at the same time.

Tailored Cycling Methods

In addition to the preset categories, a lot of people choose calorie cycling strategies that are personalized to their requirements.

This could entail modifying the length of cycles, altering the intensity of calorie variations, or incorporating particular food choices.

Customization makes it possible to take a more sustainable and individualized approach to calorie cycling, ensuring that people can stick to their diet over time.

A versatile and dynamic method of controlling calorie intake is provided by the calorie-cycling diet.

The fundamental idea is the same whether applied daily, weekly, monthly, or through personalized approaches: varying calorie intake intentionally to meet predetermined fitness and health goals. Calorie cycling should be consulted with a healthcare provider or nutritionist, as with any dietary plan, to make sure it fits your needs and other health issues.

CHAPTER FOUR

Composing Nutrient-Rich And Balanced Meals

A dietary strategy called "calorie cycling" alternates between intervals of increased and decreased calorie consumption.

To accomplish particular health and fitness goals, including weight loss, muscle gain, or increased metabolic flexibility, the aim is to carefully control calorie consumption.

Making meals that are nutrient-rich and well-balanced is a crucial component of this technique, as it guarantees that the body gets the nutrients it needs while following the calorie-cycling plan.

Focusing on including a range of nutrient-dense foods is crucial for creating balanced meals.

This consists of a variety of whole grains, lean proteins, healthy fats, and vibrant fruits and vegetables.

People can make sure they get a wide range of vitamins, minerals, and other essential nutrients required for good health by varying their meal choices.

Comprehending Macronutrients

The main and comparatively substantial sources of energy that the body needs are macronutrients.

They consist of lipids, proteins, and carbs. For calorie cycling to be efficient, it is essential to comprehend the function of each macronutrient.

The body uses fats to produce hormones and absorb nutrients, proteins are needed for muscle repair and maintenance, and carbohydrates are the preferred energy source.

It's crucial to modify the intake of these macronutrients in calorie cycling based on predetermined objectives.

For example, consuming more protein at times of increased physical activity or during phases of muscle growth may be advantageous.

On the other hand, dietary changes in fat and carbohydrate intake might be taken into account during times of decreased activity or weight loss phases.

Creating Well-Balanced Meals For Cycling Calories

Creating balanced meals for calorie cycling requires thoughtful meal planning and taking into account each person's unique nutritional requirements. Generally speaking, at particular stages of the cycle, a greater proportion of calories should be devoted to particular macronutrients.

For instance, to meet energy needs, a larger percentage of calories may come from carbohydrates on days when you work out intensely.

Lean protein sources like chicken or tofu, complex carbs like quinoa or sweet potatoes, and an assortment of vibrant veggies might make up a healthy dinner.

A tiny amount of good fats, like avocados or olive oil, improves the meal's nutritional profile even more.

Long-term success depends on modifying macronutrient ratios and portion sizes according to personal tastes and responses to the calorie cycling technique.

Example Menus

Sample meal plans offer useful information about incorporating calorie cycling into the daily diet.

These programs are made to fit individual goals by meeting predetermined macronutrient and calorie targets.

For example, a day with a larger calorie intake might have meals that have a balanced macronutrient distribution, whereas a day with fewer calories might emphasize veggies and lean meats to help with weight loss.

It's important to remember that sample meal plans should only be used as a guide; people should adjust them based on their nutritional needs, tastes, and reactions to calorie cycling.

Within the parameters of calorie cycling, flexibility can be achieved by experimenting with different meal combinations and modifying portion sizes, which encourages sustainability and adherence to the selected dietary plan.

CHAPTER FIVE

Including Exercise In The Cycling Of Calories

Any diet plan, including calorie cycling, must include exercise if it is to be successful.

The relationship between exercise and calorie cycling is examined in this section, along with how physical activity affects overall outcomes and calorie requirements.

It emphasizes how a well-planned exercise program and a cyclical diet can function in concert.

Exercise's Effect On Calorie Requirements

When engaging in calorie cycling, it is vital to comprehend how activity affects caloric requirements.

The science underlying how various forms of exercise impact energy expenditure and metabolism is covered in this subsection. If someone is doing strength training, cardiovascular exercise, or both at the same time, they can adjust their calorie cycling to fit their activity levels.

The Greatest Workouts For Cycling Calories

There are specific activities that are very beneficial for people who cycle calories. This section of the article describes workouts that will increase the efficiency of the diet by balancing its cyclical nature.

Combining these exercises can enhance fat reduction, muscle preservation, and general fitness. These exercises range from resistance training to high-intensity interval training (HIIT).

Making An Exercise Schedule

Creating an exercise regimen that works is essential for people on a calorie cycling diet.

This section offers suggestions for building an individual exercise program that adheres to the calorie cycling principles.

It addresses variables including frequency, intensity, and length and provides helpful advice for modifying the exercise regimen to fit various calorie periods.

Combining exercise with a calorie-cycling diet can increase its advantages and support a more all-encompassing strategy for fitness and health.

Realizing how activity, calorie intake, and metabolic responses interact is essential to realizing this dietary strategy's full potential.

CHAPTER SIX

Overcoming Difficulties

Adapting to energy variations is one of the main problems people have when starting a calorie-cycling diet.

It can be difficult to maintain weight loss over time since the body adjusts to regular calorie intake.

By introducing changes in calorie consumption, calorie cycling seeks to interfere with this adaption. However, adjusting to these changes can be challenging and call for careful planning.

Handling Cravings And Hunger

During the shift to a calorie-cycling diet, hunger and cravings are often encountered challenges. People may become more hungry when their calorie intake is lower, which could cause them to stray from their diet.

Making smart meal scheduling decisions, choosing nutrient-dense foods that satisfy, and drinking plenty of water are all crucial to overcoming this difficulty. Maintaining dietary adherence can also be aided by knowing the difference between genuine hunger and emotional desires.

Practical And Social Difficulties

The social side of dieting can be very difficult, particularly if you're following a calorie cycling plan.

Attending family functions, and social events, and eating out can create circumstances that make it difficult to maintain the recommended calorie intake.

Without jeopardizing the calorie cycling approach's overall effectiveness, these obstacles can be overcome by adopting useful strategies like ahead-of-time planning, communicating dietary preferences, and making wise decisions in social situations.

Maintaining Calorie Cycling Consistency

Any diet plan must be consistent to be successful, and calorie cycling is no different. Maintaining adherence requires routines that are established by individual preferences and lifestyles.

Long-term consistency can be achieved by incorporating enjoyable foods, setting realistic goals, and developing a realistic and sustainable calorie-cycling schedule. Monitoring results and adjusting as necessary can also increase the probability of continued adherence.

Troubleshooting Typical Problems

Even with meticulous preparation, people may run into common problems when following a calorie-cycling diet.

These problems may manifest as energy swings, weight loss plateaus, or challenges with precise calorie estimation. A methodical approach is needed to troubleshoot such issues, such as reevaluating calorie needs, altering macronutrient ratios, adding refeed days, or consulting a specialist.

 A more effective and long-lasting calorie cycling experience can be achieved by recognizing and proactively addressing these issues.

The calorie-cycling diet offers a dynamic and adaptable nutritional strategy that may be advantageous for people trying to control their weight.

Ensuring the successful implementation of a calorie cycling plan requires overcoming obstacles related to fluctuations in energy levels, managing hunger and cravings, navigating social situations, staying consistent, and troubleshooting common issues.

By understanding and addressing these challenges, individuals can optimize their adherence to the diet and maximize its potential benefits.

CHAPTER SEVEN

Monitoring Progress

Monitoring progress is a crucial aspect of any diet plan, including the Calorie Cycling Diet.

It involves keeping a close eye on various factors to ensure that the diet is effective and aligns with your health and fitness goals.

Tracking progress not only helps in staying motivated but also allows for adjustments to be made to optimize results.

Tracking Your Caloric Intake

One of the fundamental elements of the Calorie Cycling Diet is meticulous tracking of caloric intake. This involves recording the number of calories consumed each day and paying attention to both the quantity and quality of food. By maintaining a food diary or utilizing specialized apps, individuals can gain a comprehensive understanding of their eating habits, facilitating informed decisions about calorie adjustments.

Assessing Changes In Weight And Body Composition

A key aspect of monitoring progress on the Calorie calorie-cycling diet is regularly assessing changes in weight and body composition.

This involves stepping on the scale to track fluctuations in weight and, more importantly, measuring body fat percentage. By doing so, individuals can gain insights into the effectiveness of their diet plan, ensuring that any weight loss or gain is attributed to changes in fat mass rather than muscle mass.

Adjusting Your Approach As Needed

Flexibility is inherent in the Calorie Cycling Diet, and as progress is monitored, adjustments to the approach may be necessary.

Whether it's modifying the calorie distribution throughout the week or changing the types of foods consumed during high and low-calorie days, adapting the diet to individual needs is crucial. Regular reassessment allows for a tailored approach that aligns with specific goals and lifestyle factors.

Celebrating Milestones

Recognizing and celebrating milestones is an essential component of the Calorie Cycling Diet.

Achieving specific goals, such as reaching a target weight or seeing improvements in body composition, deserves acknowledgment.

Celebrating milestones reinforces a positive mindset, motivating individuals to stay committed to their dietary and fitness journey.

This could involve treating oneself to a small reward, sharing achievements with a support network, or setting new, challenging goals to continue the journey toward optimal health.

CHAPTER EIGHT

Success Stories

Real-Life Experiences with Calorie Cycling

Numerous individuals have shared their success stories with the Calorie Cycling Diet, highlighting its effectiveness in achieving their weight management and fitness goals.

These narratives provide insights into the diverse ways people have incorporated calorie cycling into their lifestyles and the outcomes they have experienced.

Testimonials And Transformations

Testimonials and transformations from individuals who have embraced the Calorie Cycling Diet offer a glimpse into the potential impact of this dietary strategy on both physical and mental well-being.

These personal accounts provide motivation and inspiration for those considering or currently following the Calorie Cycling Diet, showcasing the variety of paths to success and the transformative effects it can have on individuals' lives.

The calorie Cycling Diet presents a flexible and dynamic approach to managing caloric intake, potentially yielding positive outcomes for weight management and overall health. While success stories and testimonials provide anecdotal evidence of its efficacy,

individuals need to approach calorie cycling with an understanding of their unique needs and consult with healthcare professionals for personalized guidance.

Implementation Strategies

Successfully implementing a calorie cycling diet involves careful planning and consistency. Strategies may include rotating high and low-calorie days, incorporating refeed days to prevent metabolic adaptation, and adjusting calorie levels based on progress and individual response.

Regular monitoring of weight, body composition, and energy levels can help fine-tune the approach for optimal results.

Final Verdict

In conclusion, the calorie cycling diet is a nutritional strategy that aims to optimize metabolism and promote fat loss by varying calorie intake throughout the week.

While research on its long-term effectiveness is still evolving, many individuals have reported success with this approach.

As with any dietary plan, it is essential to personalize the strategy based on individual needs, preferences, and health considerations.

Recap Of Key Concepts

Key concepts in calorie cycling include varying calorie intake to prevent metabolic adaptation, setting appropriate calorie targets, paying attention to macronutrient distribution and nutrient timing, and understanding the potential benefits and drawbacks of this approach. The success of a calorie cycling diet relies on careful planning, consistency, and monitoring of individual responses.

Thoughts And Encouragement

Embarking on a calorie cycling journey requires commitment and a willingness to adapt the approach based on personal experiences. It's essential to focus on long-term health and well-being rather than short-term results.

Experimenting with different strategies, staying mindful of overall nutrition, and incorporating regular physical activity can contribute to the success of a calorie cycling diet. Remember that individual responses vary, and patience is key to achieving sustainable and positive changes in body composition and overall health.

ISBN 9798869922175
90000
9 798869 922175

THYROID TRIUMPH

Comprehensive Therapies For Optimal Thyroid Function

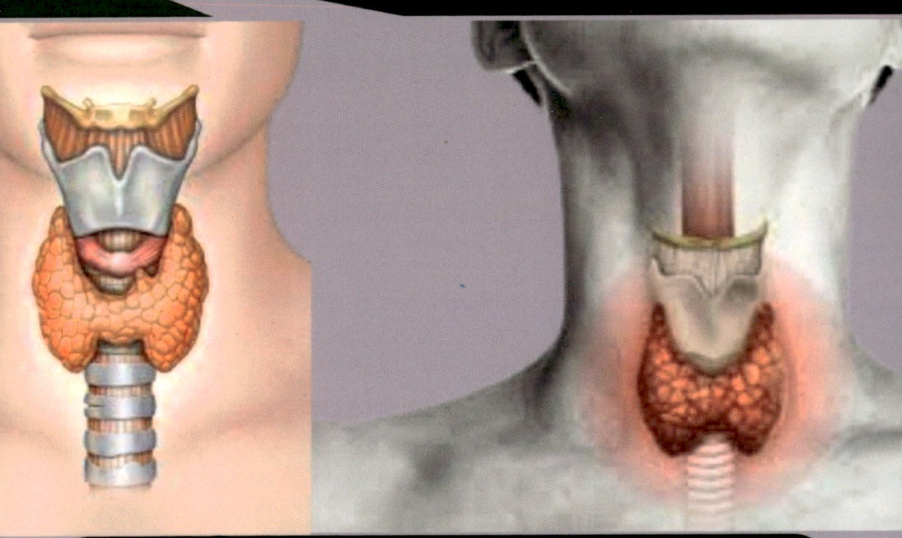

Uncover Strategies To Support Thyroid Health And Overcome Common Thyroid Disorders For A Balanced And Energized Life

DR. BRIDGET PROMISE